Table of Contents

The Mediterranean Diet - The Heart-Healthy Eating

Ultimate Guide 5

How Does the Mediterranean Diet Work Exactly? 7

What is the Mediterranean diet? 8

Can Following the Mediterranean Diet Help With

Weight Loss? 14

A Detailed Mediterranean Diet Food List to Follow:

What to Eat and Avoid 17

Olive Oil..18

Tomatoes 19

Salmon 20

Walnuts 20

Chickpeas 21

Arugula.. 22

Pomegranate 23

Lentils 24

Farro 25

Greek Yogurt... 26

A 7-Day Sample Mediterranean Diet Meal Plan . 27

Day 1 27

Day 2 28

Day 3 28

Day 4 29

Day 5 30

Day 6 31

Day 7 31

What Are the Pros and Cons of a Mediterranean

Diet?... 32

Pros 33

Cons.. 36

What Are the Potential Short- and Long-Term

Effects of a Mediterranean Diet? 39

8 tips for healthy eating 41

Saturated fat.. 48

Sugar 51

The Mediterranean Diet - The Heart-Healthy Eating Ultimate Guide

The way we think about the word "diet" today is something borne of restriction that helps you lose weight. The Mediterranean diet couldn't be further from that. Rather, it's a heart-healthy diet that includes the food staples of people who live in the region around the Mediterranean Sea, such as Greece, Croatia, and Italy.

You'll find that in their meals, they emphasize a plant-based eating approach, loaded with vegetables and healthy fats, including olive oil and omega-3 fatty acids from fish. It's a diet known for being heart-healthy. "This diet is rich in fruits and vegetables, whole grains, seafood, nuts and legumes, and olive oil". On this plan, you'll limit or avoid red meat, sugary foods, and dairy (though small amounts like yogurt and cheese are allowed).

Eating this way means you also have little room for processed fare. When you look at a plate, it should be bursting with color; traditional proteins like chicken may be more of a side dish compared with the produce packing the plate.

One thing you'll find people love about the Mediterranean diet is the allowance of moderate amounts of red wine. "Moderate" means 5 ounces (oz) or less each day for women (one glass) and no more than 10 oz daily for men (two glasses). Above all else, these meals are eaten in the company of friends and family; strong social ties are a cornerstone of healthful lives — and a healthful diet. Here, food is celebrated.

How Does the Mediterranean Diet Work Exactly?

The Mediterranean diet wasn't built as a weight loss plan — in fact, because it wasn't developed at all, but is a style of eating of a region of people that evolved naturally over centuries, there's no official way to follow it. But it's popular because it's a well-rounded approach to eating that isn't restrictive. Two of the five Blue Zones — areas where people live longer and have lower rates of disease — are located in Mediterranean cities (Ikaria, Greece and Sardinia, Italy). These places are known for having some of the lowest rates of heart disease and cancer worldwide.

What is the Mediterranean diet?

The Mediterranean diet is a way of eating based on the traditional cuisine of countries bordering the Mediterranean Sea. While there is no single definition of the Mediterranean diet, it is typically high in vegetables, fruits, whole grains, beans, nut and seeds, and olive oil.

The main components of Mediterranean diet include:

Daily consumption of vegetables, fruits, whole grains and healthy fats

Weekly intake of fish, poultry, beans and eggs

Moderate portions of dairy products

Limited intake of red meat

Other important elements of the Mediterranean diet are sharing meals with family and friends, enjoying a glass of red wine and being physically active.

Plant based, not meat based

The foundation of the Mediterranean diet is vegetables, fruits, herbs, nuts, beans and whole grains. Meals are built around these plant-based foods. Moderate amounts of dairy, poultry and eggs are also central to the Mediterranean Diet, as is seafood. In contrast, red meat is eaten only occasionally.

Healthy fats

Healthy fats are a mainstay of the Mediterranean diet. They're eaten instead of less healthy fats, such as saturated and trans fats, which contribute to heart disease.

Olive oil is the primary source of added fat in the Mediterranean diet. Olive oil provides monounsaturated fat, which has been found to lower total cholesterol and low-density lipoprotein (LDL or "bad") cholesterol levels. Nuts and seeds also contain monounsaturated fat.

Fish are also important in the Mediterranean diet. Fatty fish — such as mackerel, herring, sardines, albacore tuna, salmon and lake trout — are rich in omega-3 fatty acids, a type of polyunsaturated fat that may reduce inflammation in the body. Omega-3 fatty acids also help decrease triglycerides, reduce blood clotting, and decrease the risk of stroke and heart failure.

What Are the Potential and Known Health Benefits of the Mediterranean Diet?

The Mediterranean diet is most famous for its benefit to heart health, decreasing the risk of heart disease by, in part, lowering levels of "bad" LDL cholesterol, and reducing mortality from cardiovascular conditions. It's also been credited with a lower likelihood of certain cancers, like breast cancer, as well as conditions like Parkinson's disease and Alzheimer's disease. Emerging evidence suggests that eating this way may offer protective effects for those with and at risk for type 2 diabetes. For one, Mediterranean eating improves blood sugar control in those already diagnosed with the condition, suggesting it can be a good way to manage the disease. What's more, given those with diabetes are at increased odds for cardiovascular disease, adopting this diet can help improve their heart health, according to a paper published in April 2014 in the journal Nutrients.

Finally, people eat about nine servings of fruits and vegetables a day on a Mediterranean diet. Produce packs an array of disease-fighting antioxidants, and people who fill their diet with these foods have lower risk of disease. Yet as the National Institutes of Health points out, it's not known if it's the antioxidants or other compounds (or general healthy eating patterns) that are responsible for these advantages.

Can Following the Mediterranean Diet Help With Weight Loss?

As a traditional way of eating for many cultures worldwide, the Mediterranean diet wasn't designed for weight loss. It just so happens that one of the healthiest diets around the globe also is good for keeping your weight down.

One review, published in April 2016 in The American Journal of Medicine, looked at five research trials on overweight and obese people and found that after one year those who followed a Mediterranean diet lost as much as 11 pounds (lbs) more than low-fat eaters. (They lost between 9 and 22 lbs total and kept it off for a year.) But that same study found similar weight loss in other diets, like low-carb diets and the American Diabetes Association diet. The results suggest, the researchers say, that "there is no ideal diet for achieving sustained weight loss in overweight or obese individuals."

Yet it's an incredibly well-rounded way to lose weight that ditches gimmicks and doesn't require calorie or macronutrient counting as other diets do. And with the emphasis on healthy fat, it's satisfying, too. That said, the 2019 U.S. News & World Report Best Diets ranked the Mediterranean diet as No. 1 for Best Diets Overall and it ranks 17 in their list of Best Weight-Loss Diets. The reviewers note that it's not a slam dunk, and all depends on how you eat. Even healthy diets like the Mediterranean aren't free-for-all eating plans.

A Detailed Mediterranean Diet Food List to Follow: What to Eat and Avoid

When you're looking to start to follow the Mediterranean diet, you'll rely heavily on the following foods. While this is not a calorie-counting plan, we've included nutrition stats for your reference.

Olive Oil

Per Tablespoon Serving 120 calories, 0 grams (g) protein, 13g fat, 2g saturated fat, 10g monounsaturated fat, 0g carbohydrate, 0g fiber, 0g sugar

Benefits

Replacing foods high in saturated fats (like butter) with plant sources high in monounsaturated fatty acids, like olive oil, may help lower the risk of heart disease by 19 percent, according research — including an article published in March 2018 in the Journal of Clinical Nutrition.

Tomatoes

Per 1 cup, Chopped Serving 32 calories, 1.5g protein, 0g fat, 7g carbohydrates, 2g fiber, 5g sugar.

Benefits

It packs lycopene, a powerful antioxidant that is associated with a reduced risk of some cancers, like prostate and breast. Other components in tomatoes may help reduce the risk of blood clots, thereby protecting against cardiovascular disease, according to a review published in December 2013 in the journal Annual Review of Food Science and Technology.

Salmon

Per 3 oz Serving 133 calories, 22g protein, 5g fat,

0g carbohydrates, 0g fiber, 0g sugar

Benefits

The fatty fish is a major source of omega-3 fatty

acids. For good heart health, the American Heart

Association recommends eating at least two fish

meals per week, particularly fatty fish like salmon.

Walnuts

Per 1 oz (14 Halves) Serving 185 calories, 4g

protein, 18g fat, 2g saturated fat, 3g

monounsaturated fat, 13g polyunsaturated fat, 4g carbohydrate, 2g fiber, 1g sugar

Benefits

Rich in heart-healthy polyunsaturated fats, these nuts may also favorably impact your gut microbiome (and thus improve digestive health), as well as lower LDL cholesterol, according to a study published in May 2018 in the Journal of Nutrition.

Chickpeas

Per 1 Cup Serving 269 calories, 15g protein, 4g fat, 45g carbohydrate, 13g fiber, 8g sugar

Benefits

The main ingredient in hummus, chickpeas pack an impressive amount of fiber (more than half of a woman's 25 g daily quota), as well as iron, zinc, folate, and magnesium, according to a paper published in November 2014 in the journal Applied Physiology, Nutrition, and Metabolism. (15,16) The stats above are for a whole cup, but you only need ½ cup per day to reap the benefits.

Arugula

Per 1 Cup Serving 5 calories, 0.5g protein, 0g fat, 1g carbohydrate, 0g fiber, 0g sugar

Benefits

Leafy greens, like arugula, are eaten in abundance under this eating approach. Mediterranean-like diets that include frequent (more than six times a week) consumption of leafy greens have been shown to reduce the risk of Alzheimer's disease, according to a study published in September 2015 in the journal Alzheimer's and Dementia.

Pomegranate

Per ½ Cup Serving (arils) 72 calories, 1.5g protein, 1g fat, 16g carbohydrates, 4g fiber, 12g sugar

Benefits

This fruit, in all its bright red glory, packs powerful polyphenols that act as an antioxidant and anti-inflammatory. It's also been suggested that pomegranates may have anti-cancer properties, too.

Lentils

Per ½ Cup Serving 115 calories, 9g protein, 0g fat, 20g carbohydrate, 8g fiber, 2g sugar

Benefits

One small study published in April 2018 in the Journal of Nutrition suggested that swapping one-half of your serving of high-glycemic starches (like rice) with lentils helps lower blood glucose by 20 percent.

Farro

Per ¼ Cup (Uncooked) Serving 200 calories, 7g protein. 1.5g fat, 37g carbs, 7g fiber, 0g sugar

Benefits

Whole grains like farro are a staple of this diet. This grain offers a stellar source of satiating fiber and protein. Eating whole grains is associated with a reduced risk of a host of disease, like stroke, type 2 diabetes, heart disease, and colorectal cancer.

Greek Yogurt

Per 7-oz Container (Low-Fat Plain) 146 calories, 20g protein, 4g fat, 2g saturated fat, 1g monounsaturated fat, 0g polyunsaturated fat, 8g carbs, 0g fiber, 7g sugar

Benefits

Dairy is eaten in limited amounts, but these foods serve to supply an excellent source of calcium. Opting for low- or nonfat versions decreases the amount of saturated fat you're consuming. (25,26)

A 7-Day Sample Mediterranean Diet Meal Plan

Day 1

Breakfast: Greek yogurt topped with berries and a drizzle of honey

Snack: Handful of almonds

Lunch: Tuna on a bed of greens with a vinaigrette

Snack: Small bowl of olives

Dinner: Small chicken breast over a warm grain salad made with sautéed zucchini, tomato, and farro

Day 2

Breakfast: Whole-grain toast with a soft-boiled egg and a piece of fruit

Snack: Handful of pistachios

Lunch: Lentil salad with roasted red peppers, sun dried tomatoes, capers, and a balsamic vinaigrette

Snack: Hummus with dipping veggies

Dinner: Salmon with quinoa and sautéed garlicky greens

Day 3

Breakfast: Whipped ricotta topped with walnuts and fruit

Snack: Roasted chickpeas

Lunch: Tabouli salad with whole grain pita

Snack: Caprese skewers

Dinner: Roasted chicken, gnocchi, and a large salad with vinaigrette

Day 4

Breakfast: Fruit with a couple of slices of Brie

Snack: Cashews and dried fruit

Lunch: Vegetable soup with whole-grain roll

Snack: Tasting plate with olives, a couple slices of cheese, cucumbers, and cherry tomatoes

Dinner: White fish cooked in olive oil and garlic, spiralized zucchini, and a sweet potato

Day 5

Breakfast: Omelet made with tomatoes, fresh herbs, and olives

Snack: A couple of dates stuffed with almond butter

Lunch: A salad topped with white beans, veggies, olives, and a small piece of chicken

Snack: A peach and yogurt

Dinner: Grilled shrimp skewers with roasted Brussels sprouts

Day 6

Breakfast: Eggs scrambled with veggies and chives and topped with feta with a slice of whole-grain bread

Snack: Greek yogurt

Lunch: A quinoa bowl topped with sliced chicken, feta, and veggies

Snack: Hummus with veggies

Dinner: Grilled seafood, roasted fennel and broccoli, arugula salad, and quinoa

Day 7

Breakfast: Veggie frittata

Snack: Handful of berries

Lunch: A plate of smoked salmon, capers, lemon, whole grain crackers, and raw veggies

Snack: Mashed avocado with lemon and salt, with cucumbers for dipping

Dinner: Pasta with red sauce and mussels.

What Are the Pros and Cons of a Mediterranean Diet?

When you're deciding whether a Mediterranean Diet is right for you, consider these pros and cons:

Pros

It's easy to stick with. A diet only works if it's doable. That means everyone in your family can eat it and you can eat in this style no matter where you go (to a restaurant for dinner, to a family event). With its flavors and variety of foods that don't cut out any food group, this is one such eating plan. It is an appealing diet that one can stay with for a lifetime.

You can eat what you love. It's evident that with such a variety of whole, fresh foods available to you as options, it's easy to build meals based on the diet. And, you don't have to eliminate your favorites, either. They may just require some tweaks. For instance, rather than a sausage and pepperoni pizza, you'd choose one piled high with veggies and topped with some cheese. You can also fit in a lot of food into one meal. Filling up on fresh foods like fruits and vegetables will allow you to build volume into meals for fewer calories.

It's low in saturated fat. You're not going to feel hungry eating this way, because you can build in a variety of healthy fats. But by limiting large amounts of red or processed meats and relying heavily on monounsaturated fatty acids, like avocado, nuts, or olive oil, you'll keep saturated fat levels low. These fats don't lead to high cholesterol the same way saturated fats do. Healthful sources of fat include olive oil, fish oils, and nut-based oils.

It reduces risk of disease. A growing number of studies suggest that people who follow a Mediterranean diet are less likely to die of heart disease than people who follow a typical American diet. What's more, evidence is emerging that shows people who eat this way have a lower risk of colon cancer, prostate cancer, and some head and neck cancers, according to studies published in September 2016 in the British Journal of Cancer and in February 2018 in the Journal of Urology.

Cons

Milk is limited. There are no long-term risks to eating Mediterranean. But you may be put off if you're big on eating a lot of milk and rely on it to get all the calcium you need. You'll get to eat cheese and yogurt, but in smaller amounts. To get enough calcium in the diet without milk, one would need to eat enough yogurt and cheese, or seek nondairy calcium sources. If needed, drink skim milk. Otherwise, nondairy calcium sources include fortified almond milk, sardines, kale, and tofu made with calcium sulfate.

You still have to cap alcohol. The hallmark of a Mediterranean diet is that drinking red wine socially is thought to be one reason why the diet is so healthy. But women should still stick to one glass, and men two glasses. If you have a history of breast cancer in the family, know that any alcohol consumption raises that risk. In that case, talk to your doctor to find out what's right for you.

Fat isn't unlimited either. As with wine, it's possible to get too much of a good thing when it comes to healthy fats. The American Heart Association points out that while the Mediterranean diet meets heart-healthy diet limits for saturated fat, your total fat consumption could be greater than the daily recommended amount if you aren't careful.

That's 65 g per day.

You have to find time to cook. While you don't

have to spend hours in your kitchen, you will need

to cook because the diet is all about working with

delicious fresh food. You may have a learning

curve as you build these skills.

What Are the Potential Short- and Long-Term Effects of a Mediterranean Diet?

As has become obvious, there are numerous potential benefits from adopting a Mediterranean diet. Over the long term, these health effects may be more pronounced and can include better brain health by slowing cognitive decline and lowering risk of Alzheimer's disease and other dementias.

It also may help stave off chronic diseases, like heart disease and type 2 diabetes, as well as act protectively against certain cancers. The diet is also a boon to mental health, as it's associated with reduced odds of depression. There's even some data to suggest it can be supportive in relieving symptoms of arthritis, according to a paper published in April 2018 in the journal Frontiers in Psychology.

In the short term, you may lose a modest amount of weight over a year span and are likely to keep it off it you continue to eat following the diet. If eating in the Mediterranean style prompts you to consume more fruits and vegetables, you'll not only feel better physically, but your mental health will get a lift, too. Research shows that people who eat more raw fruits and veggies (particularly dark leafy greens like spinach, fresh berries, and cucumber) have fewer symptoms of depression, a better mood, and more life satisfaction.

8 tips for healthy eating

These 8 practical tips cover the basics of healthy eating and can help you make healthier choices.

The key to a healthy diet is to eat the right amount of calories for how active you are so you balance the energy you consume with the energy you use.

If you eat or drink more than your body needs, you'll put on weight because the energy you do not use is stored as fat. If you eat and drink too little, you'll lose weight.

You should also eat a wide range of foods to make sure you're getting a balanced diet and your body is receiving all the nutrients it needs.

It's recommended that men have around 2,500 calories a day (10,500 kilojoules). Women should have around 2,000 calories a day (8,400 kilojoules).

Most adults in the UK are eating more calories than they need and should eat fewer calories.

1. Base your meals on higher fibre starchy carbohydrates

Starchy carbohydrates should make up just over a third of the food you eat. They include potatoes, bread, rice, pasta and cereals.

Choose higher fibre or wholegrain varieties, such as wholewheat pasta, brown rice or potatoes with their skins on.

They contain more fibre than white or refined starchy carbohydrates and can help you feel full for longer.

Try to include at least 1 starchy food with each main meal. Some people think starchy foods are fattening, but gram for gram the carbohydrate they contain provides fewer than half the calories of fat.

Keep an eye on the fats you add when you're cooking or serving these types of foods because that's what increases the calorie content – for example, oil on chips, butter on bread and creamy sauces on pasta.

2. Eat lots of fruit and veg

It's recommended that you eat at least 5 portions of a variety of fruit and veg every day. They can be fresh, frozen, canned, dried or juiced.

Getting your 5 A Day is easier than it sounds. Why not chop a banana over your breakfast cereal, or swap your usual mid-morning snack for a piece of fresh fruit?

A portion of fresh, canned or frozen fruit and vegetables is 80g. A portion of dried fruit (which should be kept to mealtimes) is 30g.

A 150ml glass of fruit juice, vegetable juice or smoothie also counts as 1 portion, but limit the amount you have to no more than 1 glass a day as these drinks are sugary and can damage your teeth.

3. Eat more fish, including a portion of oily fish

Fish is a good source of protein and contains many

vitamins and minerals.

Aim to eat at least 2 portions of fish a week,

including at least 1 portion of oily fish.

Oily fish are high in omega-3 fats, which may help

prevent heart disease.

Oily fish include:

salmon

trout

herring

sardines

pilchards

mackerel

Non-oily fish include:

haddock

plaice

coley

cod

tuna

skate

hake

You can choose from fresh, frozen and canned, but remember that canned and smoked fish can be high in salt.

Most people should be eating more fish, but there are recommended limits for some types of fish.

4. Cut down on saturated fat and sugar

Saturated fat

You need some fat in your diet, but it's important to pay attention to the amount and type of fat you're eating.

There are 2 main types of fat: saturated and unsaturated. Too much saturated fat can increase the amount of cholesterol in the blood, which increases your risk of developing heart disease.

On average, men should have no more than 30g of saturated fat a day. On average, women should have no more than 20g of saturated fat a day.

Children under the age of 11 should have less saturated fat than adults, but a low-fat diet is not suitable for children under 5.

Saturated fat is found in many foods, such as:

fatty cuts of meat

sausages

butter

hard cheese

cream

cakes

biscuits

lard

pies

Try to cut down on your saturated fat intake and choose foods that contain unsaturated fats instead, such as vegetable oils and spreads, oily fish and avocados.

For a healthier choice, use a small amount of vegetable or olive oil, or reduced-fat spread instead of butter, lard or ghee.

When you're having meat, choose lean cuts and cut off any visible fat.

All types of fat are high in energy, so they should only be eaten in small amounts.

Sugar

Regularly consuming foods and drinks high in sugar increases your risk of obesity and tooth decay.

Sugary foods and drinks are often high in energy (measured in kilojoules or calories), and if consumed too often can contribute to weight gain. They can also cause tooth decay, especially if eaten between meals.

Free sugars are any sugars added to foods or drinks, or found naturally in honey, syrups and unsweetened fruit juices and smoothies.

This is the type of sugar you should be cutting down on, rather than the sugar found in fruit and milk.

Many packaged foods and drinks contain surprisingly high amounts of free sugars.

Free sugars are found in many foods, such as:

sugary fizzy drinks

sugary breakfast cereals

cakes

biscuits

pastries and puddings

sweets and chocolate

alcoholic drinks

Food labels can help. Use them to check how much sugar foods contain.

More than 22.5g of total sugars per 100g means the food is high in sugar, while 5g of total sugars or less per 100g means the food is low in sugar. Get tips on cutting down on sugar in your diet

5. Eat less salt: no more than 6g a day for adults

Eating too much salt can raise your blood pressure. People with high blood pressure are more likely to develop heart disease or have a stroke.

Even if you do not add salt to your food, you may still be eating too much.

About three-quarters of the salt you eat is already in the food when you buy it, such as breakfast cereals, soups, breads and sauces.

Use food labels to help you cut down. More than 1.5g of salt per 100g means the food is high in salt.

Adults and children aged 11 and over should eat no more than 6g of salt (about a teaspoonful) a day. Younger children should have even less.

Get tips on cutting down on salt in your diet

6. Get active and be a healthy weight

As well as eating healthily, regular exercise may help reduce your risk of getting serious health conditions. It's also important for your overall health and wellbeing.

Being overweight or obese can lead to health conditions, such as type 2 diabetes, certain cancers, heart disease and stroke. Being underweight could also affect your health.

Most adults need to lose weight by eating fewer calories.

If you're trying to lose weight, aim to eat less and be more active. Eating a healthy, balanced diet can help you maintain a healthy weight.

Check whether you're a healthy weight by using the BMI healthy weight calculator.

Start the NHS weight loss plan, a 12-week weight loss guide that combines advice on healthier eating and physical activity.

If you're underweight, see underweight adults. If you're worried about your weight, ask your GP or a dietitian for advice.

7. Do not get thirsty

You need to drink plenty of fluids to stop you getting dehydrated. The government recommends drinking 6 to 8 glasses every day. This is in addition to the fluid you get from the food you eat.

All non-alcoholic drinks count, but water, lower fat milk and lower sugar drinks, including tea and coffee, are healthier choices.

Try to avoid sugary soft and fizzy drinks, as they're high in calories. They're also bad for your teeth.

Even unsweetened fruit juice and smoothies are high in free sugar.

Your combined total of drinks from fruit juice, vegetable juice and smoothies should not be more than 150ml a day, which is a small glass.

Remember to drink more fluids during hot weather or while exercising.

8. Do not skip breakfast

Some people skip breakfast because they think it'll help them lose weight.

But a healthy breakfast high in fibre and low in fat, sugar and salt can form part of a balanced diet, and can help you get the nutrients you need for good health.

A wholegrain lower sugar cereal with semi-skimmed milk and fruit sliced over the top is a tasty and healthier breakfast.

The Mediterranean diet is one of the healthy eating plans recommended by the Dietary Guidelines for Americans to promote health and prevent chronic disease.

It is also recognized by the World Health Organization as a healthy and sustainable dietary pattern and as an intangible cultural asset by the United National Educational, Scientific and Cultural Organization.

www.ingramcontent.com/pod-product-compliance
Lightning Source LLC
Chambersburg PA
CBHW070807250726
48662CB00004B/2012

* 9 7 9 8 6 3 2 5 3 8 6 0 2 *